*a guide to holistic discovery*

# 22 WAYS TO HEAL YOU

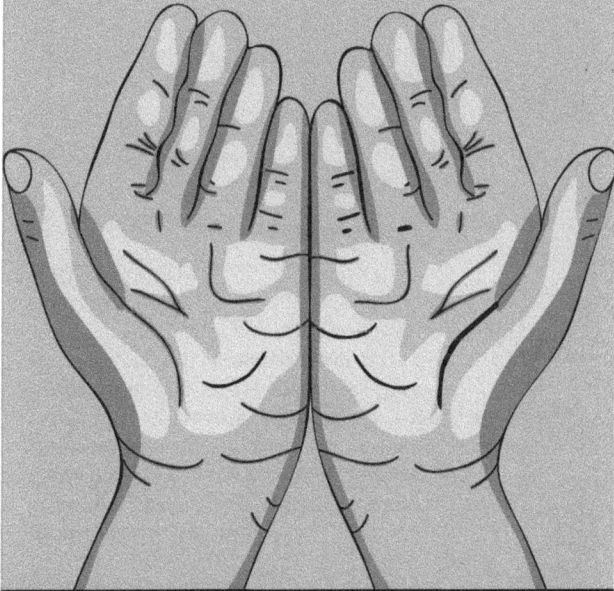

FELICIA GUY-LYNCH

# Dedication

To all those striving to heal and maintain salvation

# Aromatherapy

Burn incense.
Open the window and just vibe.

*check out: gonesh.com*

# Be Assertive

Speak the truth, even if your voice trembles

*check within*

# Bentonite Clay and Psyllium Husk

*consult a health professional*

*What are some benefits?*

The bentonite clay absorbs toxins and the psyllium husk scrubs out the corners of your intestines. This encourages the:

- Removal of plastics and heavy metals
- Reversal of radiation exposure
- Alleviation of symptoms associated with irritable bowel syndrome (IBS)

# Colon Hydrotherapy

It is commonly referred to as a colonic irrigation or colon cleansing. It's similar to an enema but uses more liquid along with special herbs, enzymes or probiotics to accentuate the healing process.

Some of the benefits are that it stimulates bowel movement, increases your chances of fertility and helps to maintain a healthy pH level for your blood.

*check out: yurielkaim.com*

# Colour

Yes! Get a colouring book and feed your inner youth!

*check out: staples.com*

# Embrace Minimalism

Or at least try to by finding what you can donate or sell
to create more space for yourself.
What you no longer need can be treasured by another.

*check out: becomingminimalist.com*

# Enema

*What is it and what are the benefits?*

- An enema is a procedure that involves injecting a liquid or gas, into the rectum through the anus to either administer medication or flush out fecal matter
- It can help with treating ulcerative colitis, alleviating severe constipation and assisting medical professionals with giving a diagnosis

*check out: badgut.org*

# Exercise

Health is wealth.
The real bag is peace of mind.
Put in some sweat equity.

*check out: thehealthy.com*

# Express

The more you repress and suppress how you really feel,
the more you stress out your soul.
Process.
Write it out.
Talk it out.
Repeat.

*call a friend. meet up somewhere*

# Fiber Intake

*What are the different types?*

**Cellulose** - insoluble fiber found in vegetables like cabbage that bind to other food particles to assist with bowel movement

**Inulin** - soluble fiber derived from chicory root found naturally in wheat like barley. It leaves you feeling fuller for longer by slowing down digestion

**Pectin** - soluble fiber found in vegetables like strawberries help reduce the glycemic response of foods by stalling glucose absorption. In other words, no sugar spikes

**Beta-Glucans** - a gel-forming type of soluble fiber found in foods like reishi mushrooms that easily gets broken down by the gut flora

**Psyllium** - a prebiotic, soluble fiber found in high-fiber cereals that help relieve constipation by softening bowels to help it pass

**Lignin** - an insoluble fiber that's part of the cell wall structure in plants such as avocados that may help to reduce the risk of developing colon cancer

**Resistant Starch** - a type of fiber found in legumes and beans that passes through the large intestine, protecting the GI tract from harmful bacteria

# Fiber Intake

*What are the different types?*

**Cellulose** - insoluble fiber found in vegetables like cabbage that bind to other food particles to assist with bowel movement

**Inulin** - soluble fiber derived from chicory root found naturally in wheat like barley. It leaves you feeling fuller for longer by slowing down digestion

**Pectin** - soluble fiber found in vegetables like strawberries help reduce the glycemic response of foods by stalling glucose absorption. In other words, no sugar spikes

**Beta Glucans** - a gel-forming type of soluble fiber found in foods like reishi mushrooms that easily gets broken down by the gut flora

**Psyllium** - a prebiotic, soluble fiber found in high-fiber cereals that help relieve constipation by softening bowels to help it pass

**Lignin** - an insoluble fiber that's part of the cell wall structure in plants such as avocados that may help to reduce the risk of developing colon cancer

**Resistant Starch** - a type of fiber found in legumes and beans that passes through the large intestine, protecting the GI tract from harmful bacteria

# Guidance

Get trusted, professional help to unpack, make sense of,
cope and overcome past trauma.
You are not your mistakes.

*check out: therapytribe.com*

# Have Faith

It's been a trying time for everyone.
You're not alone.
Be honest about your values and why they
are important to you.

*check within*

# Introspect

Progression is way more important
then pretending to be perfect.
Accept where you are.
Take a step back if you need to.

*check the barometer of your self-awareness*

# Ionic
# Foot Bath

*What is it and what are the benefits?*

- This process gives the hydrogen in the water a positive charge. The positive charge attracts the negatively charged toxins in your body. The ions in the foot bath water hold a charge that enables them to bind to heavy metals and toxins in your body. This allows the toxins to be pulled out through the bottoms of your feet

| Color of the Water | Area of the Body Represented/Detoxified |
| --- | --- |
| Black | liver |
| Black Flecks | heavy metals |
| Blue | kidney |
| Brown | liver, tobacco, cellular debris |
| Green | gallbladder |
| Orange | joints |
| Red Flecks | cellular debris, blood clot material |
| Yellow | kidney, bladder, urinary tract, female/prostate area |
| Cheesy | candidas, fungal infections, most likely yeast |
| Foam | lymphatic drainage, mucus |
| Oil Floating | fat |

*check out: healthline.com*

# Lemon and Ginger

*What are some benefits?*

- Fights infection with its combined anti-inflammatory, anti-bacterial, anti-fungal, anti-diabetic, anti-cancer and anti-viral properties
- Reduces nausea
- Optimizes thyroid health

*check out: emilykylenutrition.com*

# Prognosis

Don't get into the trap of self-diagnosis.
Follow up with a health professional.
Make adjustments to your lifestyle on a need basis.

*call your doctor to book an appointment*

# Refrain

You can't purge out if you keep
letting the wrong energy in.
Learn to govern yourself.
It's the only time you're really free.

*keep your loins in check*

# Release

Everyone is a villain in someone's story.
How can you heal the mind and body when you
consciously choose to nurse poison within your heart?
Free up yourself.

*check out: theforgivenessproject.com*

# Self-Care

You can only tend to people and things you love as
good as you tend to yourself.
The first law of nature is self-preservation.
It's not the same as being selfish.

*check out: verywellmind.com*

# Share

Knowledge is subject to change.
You'd be surprised what you can learn from
staying open-minded.
Make sure your source of information is
credible and edifying.

*check your cypher*

# Zone In

Don't forget your blindspot too!

*check your mind's eye*